FOREWORD

Whether this is your first step i
you're a long-time devotee of
power to change people's lives. I happen

At the age of 21, I was told that I would not live to see 30 because of a serious autoimmune disease. My only chance at survival? Over 15 months of grueling, heartbreaking chemotherapy. It was a long-hard battle—one that I still face every day. And, I couldn't do it without my Young Living Essential Oils.

I'm a long way past 30 (or maybe I've just turned 29 a few times), but I have to say this new lease on life inspired me to make a difference. The past two decades I've devoted myself to the cause of education. But I'm not talking about the make-you-snore-take-a-test-and-forget kind of learning. (Obviously, that has its place. I think…) I'm talking about real knowledge that people can use right away. I'm talking about the self-empowering kind of education, the kind that really frees you to take your life, your health, and your future into your own hands.

In fact, this volume and its many companion volumes are the perfect way to get not only acquainted with essential oils and their many uses, but to do something with them right away. Today, in fact. Every year, my team and I search for the best, most updated information and scientific studies to continue building practical education tools for people to use. It has become an ongoing labor of love and a personal passion. I firmly believe that education is the key to improving the health and lives of everyone in this world.

My company, Life Science Publishing, has been around since Young Living's beginning. While I wasn't there when the doors opened, I certainly know the daily struggles that come with being an entrepreneur. There are constant ups and downs. I can't say they are easy, but I would say they are worth it. I have turned to great mentors in my life, and I believe we can all learn from someone who has been in our shoes before.

Now, I'm not here to sell you oils. I'm here to invite you to learn the simple, practical ways they can make a difference in your life—and the lives of the loved ones around you. I'm here to help you get introduced to oils and help you learn how to put them into your own homemade recipes and solutions.

I would love to say we've met, but if all you know of me is the picture in this book, I hope to meet you soon! I've been told that my energy and passion are contagious. If that's the case, I hope you catch them both…

Love. Learn. Share.

xoxo

Troie Battles

Troie Storms-Battles

FOREWARD BY CO-AUTHOR
Connie McDanel

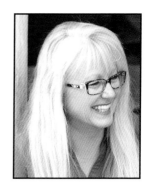

By the year 2000, I had been teaching elementary children for many years. I witnessed and was puzzled by the ever-increasing number of children crossing my classroom door presenting symptoms of allergies and asthma. Coincidentally I began a graduate degree program in special education, as almost one third of my student population was labeled "at risk," having needs ranging from attention deficit disorder (ADD) to cognitive learning disabilities.

These diagnoses, at present, are all too common place. Thus, I began to read publications from the medical, psychological, and scientific communities about the alarming statistics concerning child neural-developmental issues. Many studies implicated the role of environmental exposures from pervasive, synthetic chemicals, such as pesticides and herbicides on our food to the exposure of respiratory triggers, such as bleach in cleaners and synthetic fragrances. In fact, the studies initiated a new field of interest, pediatric environmental health. Even more alarming to me was our apparent societal complacency to recognize everyday household chemical exposures as a link and our unwillingness to take action against these neural and hormonally disruptive chemicals. The good news is we can reduce exdposure with simple changes in our consumer purchasing choices and habits. I found informing others how to create a healthier classroom environment and a healing home became a deep conviction within me; especially since my own children were young and still developing. This conviction has further developed into this series, Aroma Home, Aroma Clean, and now Aroma Family.

With Aroma Family, we are excited to share some of our favorite DIY recipes as so many families love getting back to the way grandma did it and they want to assure for themselves the quality of the ingredients in their home products. Enjoy these recipes and add your own on the back pages.

FOREWARD BY CO-AUTHOR
Katherine T. Fuller

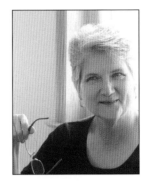

Being a scientist has taught me not to be afraid to try new things; it's okay to be creative and inventive. Cooking is a science, for example, and I love to cook. We can follow a basic recipe and produce the acceptable culinary product. Alternatively, with trial and error, it's fun to tweak that recipe to see if an even better outcome can be brought to the table. This is true with essential oils, too. I view working with essential oils as a journey. Like many of you, I began with a small cadre of oils, such as Peppermint, Lavender, Lemon, Thieves, Purification, and a few others. When I had a question about the use of an oil, I consulted the Essential Oils Desk Reference (www.discoverlsp.com) with its wealth of information and it provided clarity.

After working with essential oils for the past decade, I have become comfortable in producing my own blends to address targeted issues. My inner scientist loves to experiment with essential oils in DIY products that I know are good for me, my husband, and our beagle. Purchasing an oil and leaving it locked in a cabinet is a self-imposed roadblock in one's essential oil journey. Some oils are expensive, while others are very reasonably priced. Considering a 15 ml bottle contains approximately 200 drops of Mother Nature's potent goodness, a little bit goes a long way. The recipes provided in AROMA FAMILY are mindful of the purity and potency Young Living oils provide. One drop of a pure "14-carat" oil like Sandalwood, sparingly used, goes a long way and its benefits; priceless. By the way because of Essential Rewards, I rarely purchase these more expensive oils. I earn them with Essential Reward points. So, I challenge and invite you to discover your inner scientist as you learn to freelance your own essential oil DIY products.   –Katherine T. Fuller, B.S., M.S.-

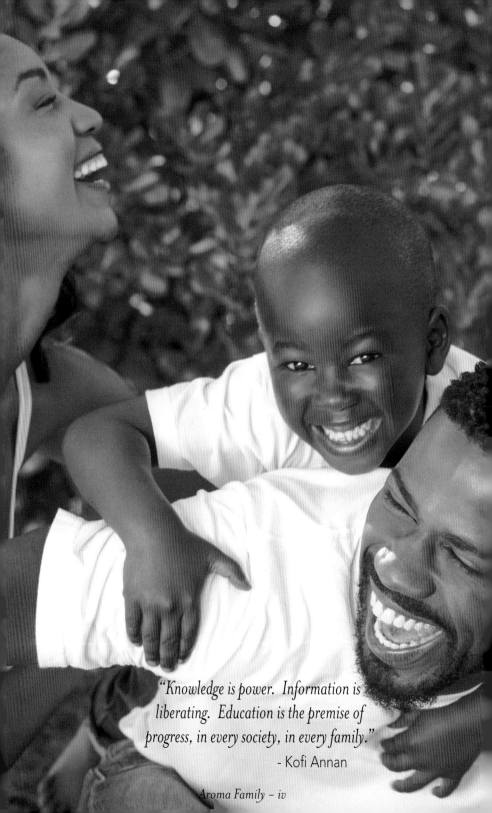

"Knowledge is power. Information is
liberating. Education is the premise of
progress, in every society, in every family."
                                        - Kofi Annan

TABLE OF CONTENTS

FAMILY

The skin is our first line of defense; yet when it comes to toxic ingredients, it is not as protective as we would like for it to be. Fact is, what we place on our skin does matter, as harmful substances can be absorbed into the bloodstream. Consider our present use of nicotine skin patches to address smoking cessation and birth control patches as a family planning measure. In 2005, the Environmental Working Group (EWG) published a combination of two scientific studies that found 287 toxic substances present in umbilical cord blood of newborns. Of the 287 toxins, 217 were neurotoxic, and 208 were known to damage growth development leading to birth defects. These statistics are concerning, even frightening, and they emphasize the critical decision-making involved in what we place on our bodies daily.

Building awareness and changing buying habits may seem daunting; however, when we become informed, then we can strategically make decisions and develop new routines. In Aroma Home we ask you to consider how our homes could potentially be exposing us to more harm than good with the personal care and cleaning product choices we are making. The "Going Green" concept stops short of the goal, since it does not address the accumulation of toxins within our bodies, nor do "green" products provide any added health supportive benefits beyond the cleaning action.

An aroma home transcends the concept of "beyond green" by producing benefits that inspire families to go a step further creating a healing home. A healing home supports an environment conducive to rejuvenation and restoration, leaving feelings of purpose, joy and gratitude.

So how does one begin changing their purchasing habits and choices of products?

A product that you place all over your body, but do not wash off, automatically is a consideration for change. (Lotions, hand sanitizers, perfumes, bug sprays, etc.).

A product that covers areas with a significant blood vessel to skin surface ratio becomes a second priority. The scalp, arm pits, and genitalia fit in this second priority. (Shampoos, conditioners, bath gels, shave creams, etc.)

Our bodies naturally cleanse, so remain calm. We do not need to overreact, but we do need to become aware and reduce our daily exposures. It becomes a more urgent topic as these exposures accumulate with time. So, our goal is to reduce the exposures and keep our cleansing mechanisms working optimally.

Is it possible to create a home environment where we feel restored, rejuvenated, and thereby acquire greater vitality?

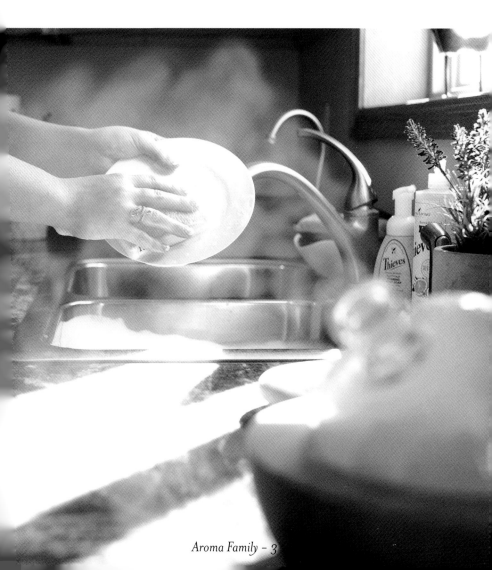

STEPS TO CREATING A HEALING HOME, AN AROMA HOME

1. **BECOME AWARE** of how toxins affect our vitality. Use the Aroma Home Planning Guide.

2. **ELIMINATE** risks with product replacement. Use the Aroma Home Planning Guide.

3. **CHOOSE** products with additional HEALTH SUPPORTIVE BENEFITS, going beyond green from the Young Living product guide.

4. **CLEANSE** accumulated toxic residues from the body following the guidelines in the Essential Oil Desk Reference.

5. **IMPLEMENT** Aroma Home and Aroma Clean Monthly Product Planning (The Young Living Essential Rewards customer loyalty program can help you acquire greater value for your dollar)

It is important that we become the CEO of our own health. By doing so, we automatically become the CEO of our family's health. We don't have to be perfect consumers; however, we have to strategically choose our household and personal care products wisely. This is how we go about reducing toxic exposures, finding alternative replacements, and in the case of AROMA FAMILY, making our own reliable DIY products with essential oils.

Top Products of Concerns:
1. Any product used to clean the home
2. Personal care products
(Bubble bath, of particular concern for children)
3. Any product we do not wash off (lotions, after shave, sunscreens, bug repellents, etc.)
4. Shampoos and conditioners (Baby shampoos, of particular concern for children)
5. Beauty products
6. Hand soaps and hand sanitizers
7. Deodorant (underarms, genitalia have high blood vessel to skin surface ratio)
8. Baby wipes, hand wipes, car wipes
9. Fragrance products vs natural aromas
10. Petroleum-based products

Feeling a bit overwhelmed; then find a full disclosure company whose products present no hidden ingredients. This is a company that you can trust. Alternatively, discover the fun and joy in making your own DIY or Do-It-Yourself household and personal care products. You are in control, you decide the ingredients, you decide the scents; you become the CEO of your health and wellness.

This is what Aroma Family is all about. Having some fun, while making an impact on your family with the reduction of toxic exposures and with the creation of your own DIY products and recipes (Burnes, Deborah).

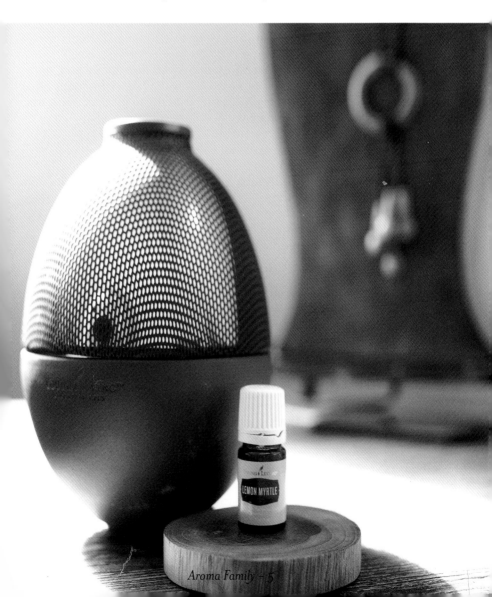

WHY SHOULD WE CARE?
10 CONCERNS

1) Between cosmetics, perfumes, personal care products and feminine hygiene products, women in the U.S. apply an average of 168 chemicals to their faces and bodies every day (EWG).

2) In 2000, cleaning products were responsible for nearly 10% of all toxic exposures reported to U.S. Poison Control Centers. **Of the total, 120,434 exposures involved children under the age of six (Organic Consumers).**

3) **Fragrances** are volatile compounds, often derived from petroleum, that linger in the air contributing to poor air quality. The EPA acknowledges that fragrances contribute to a host of problems including **headaches, dizziness, fatigue, and forgetfulness (Bridges).**

4) The National Institute of Occupational Safety and Health has found **one third** of the substances used in the fragrance industry are **toxic.** Their presence protected by **"trade secrets"** on the labeling which is used by **nondisclosure companies** (Bridges).

5) Researchers in the scientific community have linked asthma risk to frequent use of fragranced products, particularly those that are aerosol-based (Bridges).

6) Endocrine-disrupting compounds (EDCs) can act to:
   a. **Reduce the production of hormones in endocrine glands**
   b. **Affect the release of hormones from endocrine glands**
   c. **Copy or counteract the action of hormones at target tissues, or**
   d. **Speed up the metabolism of hormones reducing their action** (Greenfacts)

7) An Environmental Health Perspectives study indicates the following contained EDCs: cleaners, laundry and dishwashing soaps, stain removers, shampoos, conditioners, face lotions, cleansers, toothpastes, deodorants, cosmetics, anything vinyl, dryer sheets, air fresheners, perfumes, sunscreens (webmed.com).

8) Antibacterial agent triclosan, an EPA identified pesticide, has been banned by the FDA from soaps; however, it is still allowed in a leading U.S. toothpaste, cosmetics, athletic clothing, and cleaning products. A 2016 review of studies from the University of California San Diego reported that

triclosan may contribute to antibiotic resistance and disrupt hormones and immunity; it also has been linked to tumors in mice (consumer reports).

9) **Sodium Lauryl Sulfate or Sodium Laureth Sulfate (SLS)** is used as a foaming agent in shampoo, shower gel, liquid soap, baby products, bubble bath, and other products. The Journal of the American College of Toxicology states SLS has a "degenerative effect on cell membranes because it denatures membrane proteins." It also has the ability to be absorbed across the skin and it is frequently disguised in semi-natural cosmetics as a "coconut-based ingredient." Its presence in consumer soaps is a reason to DIY your own soap products (kindsoap.com).

10) The U.S. is at risk of falling behind other countries in addressing safety and public health concerns. If the U.S. wants to maintain its competitiveness in the world market, it needs to stop producing products that contain toxic chemicals. *"Made in the USA should be a guarantee, not a warning." (ewg.org).*

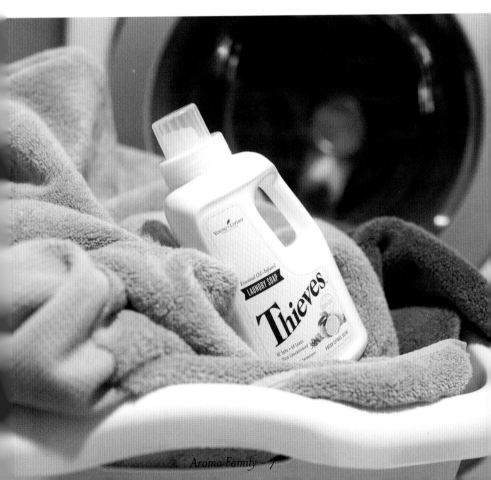

The good news, Young Living Essential Oils is a full disclosure company that guarantees the purity and quality of the essential oils found in all of its products that can replace conventional household and personal care products, reducing toxic exposures in our homes. Additionally, essential oils cleanse and work with the body to maintain and balance our systems. Essential oils present added benefits that we desire in household and personal care products used by our families.

Essential oils can be purchased from multiple companies online, at farmer's markets, and through local co-ops. However, not all brands of essential oils are the same, not even those marketed as organic. To illustrate, lavender oil provides an excellent example to differentiate between Young Living's lavender oil and those prepared and promoted by others in the essential oil industry. Companies, other than Young Living, must combine oils from several types of lavender other than pure lavender. The supply of pure lavender, *Lavendula angustifolia*, cannot keep up with the demand for pure lavender by the aromatherapy/cosmetic industry. As a consequence, other essential oil companies market an adulterated lavender oil which is a blend of pure lavender with lavendin and spike lavender. Lavender, of course, is a beautiful, multi-use oil, often topically applied to the skin. Is there a concern with an oil that is not true to its purity? An adulterated lavender oil extended by the presence of lavendin oil, high in camphor content; this would be very problematic for skin that has been burned or scraped, as the camphor would painfully exacerbate injured tissue.

When contemplating the value of an Aroma Home, therapeutic grade must be the goal. Young Living's promise to consumers is the delivery of oils as close to Mother Nature's design as possible. This is why Young Living maintains its own seed lines and follows strict certification of plant lines with scientific research, field studies, and by maintaining university partnerships, and on-site certification. Plants are grown and cultivated on Young Living farms and cooperatives utilizing optimal growing conditions, including consideration of soil type and other planting practices. The low temperature, low-pressure distillation promotes the chemical integrity of an oil. Each oil must pass Young Living's stringent testing protocol to insure bioactive constituents are not compromised. Not only does Young Living maintain its own labs for analysis, third party audits are utilized to verify that international purity and potency standards are met and surpassed. We have found no other company that goes to such measures to obtain, farm, harvest, distill, and educate for the purpose of fostering stewardship for nature's gifts of essential oils. This is why each Young Living oil is Mother Nature or therapeutic grade (Young Living website 2012).

Essential oils work with us in multiple ways and this addresses why pure oils are best. Oils are small carbon-based (organic) molecules with unique phenolic or terpenoid attachments off of the carbon structure. As carbon-based molecules, this is significant because of the chemical cleansing ability of carbon atoms/molecules. If you own a fish tank in which you use a filter system; then you probably are using an activated carbon filter to clean the water. Carbon is excellent for the removal of wastes and pollutants. Essential oils are classified as organic lipids. Lipid-based tissues of the human body include our skin and the brain, for example. Even our three trillion cell membranes, the outer definition of a cell, are lipid-based with imbedded protein molecules dotting the membrane landscape.

Critically pertinent to the cleansing nature of oils, besides their carbon core, are the unique phenolic or terpenoid attachment molecules. Chemically-speaking, lipids like lipids, meaning lipids have the ability to interact with each other. This allows essential oils to diffuse across lipid-based barriers, such as our skin or our cell membranes. Diffusion is an energetically passive transport system, in which molecules move based on their concentration gradients. An essential oil topically applied to one's skin is in higher concentration on the outside of the skin compared to the inside of the skin, so the oil moves from high to low across the skin barrier. This is true of cell membranes as well, as oils can move high to low across the membrane barrier.

At the cellular level, the unique phenolic or terpenoid molecules associated with each oil may also interact with cell membrane protein receptors. Membrane protein receptors are similar to address mailboxes lining your city street. Only your mail is meant for your mailbox because your addresses match. Membrane receptor proteins allow only certain molecular shapes to dock with them and depending upon the unique phenolic or terpenoid constituents of an oil, the oil may dock (go into the mailbox) of a cellular protein receptor. In the chemistry of biology, shape is everything. Essential oils have molecular shapes that connect with cellular protein receptors. Just as mail is communication for us, these shapes and receptors serve as communication for the cell.

"Essential oils are therapeutically multifaceted.
The components within an essential oil may produce a different
reaction in one person than in another;
depending on the availability of receptor sites."
-Dr. Jane Buckle

BASIC GUIDELINES FOR USE OF ESSENTIAL OILS IN THE FAMILY

STORAGE	CAUTIONARY USE	Application
Store in amber bottles	Oils rich in menthol (peppermint) are not suggested to be used on neck or throat area of children < 18 months	Topically apply oils to bottoms of feet or use in bath water, no more than 10 drops
Capped tightly	Citrus oils, Bergamot are photosensitive. Stay out of sun, 1-2 days after application or cover usage area.	Direct inhalation of oils, up to 10-15 times daily
Keep in cool location, out of light	Keep essential oils from eyes and ears. Do not touch eyes, glasses, or contact lenses.	Inhalation of oils not recommended for asthmatics
Keep out of reach of children	People exhibiting chronic, pre-existing health conditions (epilepsy, hypertension, i.e.) should consult physician before use. Particular caution with high ketone oils such as, Basil, Rosemary, Sage, and Tansy oils.	Before internal ingestion, try dilution in Blue Agave, Yacon syrups, or olive or coconut oils, rice milk
Keep vegetable oil on hand for dilution (V-6 Oil complex, other veggie oils)	Pregnant women or people exhibiting allergies should consult their physicians prior to use. Dilution of oils with a vegetable-based oil suggested. Skin patch test on the underside of the arm for 30 minutes warranted. Use common sense.	Reactions to essential oils, topically or by ingestion, may be delayed 2-3 days after use

Chemical Sensitivities & Allergies: Those with extra-sensitive skin, who begin using ultra-pure essential oils, will experience rashes or reactions. This may occur with an undiluted spice, conifer, or the citrus oils. An oil may react with petroleum-based residues which remain in fatty tissue from personal care products that have leached into the skin.

Before beginning with oils, try a skin test. Spot test on an area such as the inside of the forearm at the elbow. Apply one oil or blend at one time. If layering a new oil, allow 3-5 minutes to assess for a reaction, before testing a different oil. If you express a sensitivity, then follow the dilution protocol.

DILUTE:

- Dilute 1-3 drops of essential oil in ½ teaspoon of Young Living's V-6 Vegetable Oil Complex, massage oil, or any pure vegetable oil such as almond, coconut, avocado, or olive. More dilution may be required.
- Reduce the number of oils used at any time.
- Use single oils or oil blends one at a time.
- Reduce the amount of oil used.
- Reduce the frequency of application.
- Drink more purified or distilled water.
- **UTILIZE NATURAL HOUSEHOLD CLEANING SOLUTIONS TO REDUCE DAILY CHEMICAL EXPOSURES**

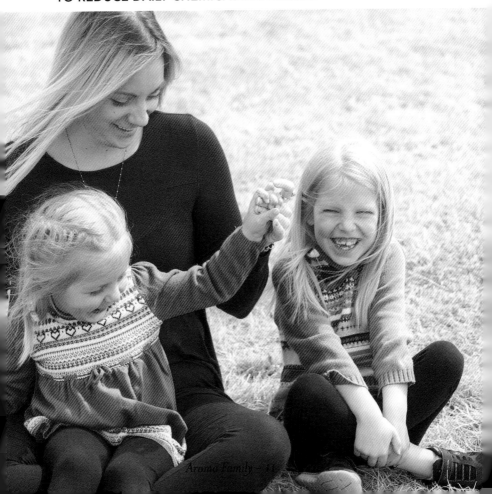

NATURAL HOUSEHOLD CLEANING NECESSITIES

NATURAL **CLEANING** SUBSTANCE	**CLEANING** RATIONALE	**CLEANSING** ESSENTIAL OILS BY YOUNG LIVING
Baking Soda (Sodium Bicarbonate)	Slightly alkaline (base) in pH which neutralizes acids and denatures proteins. Makes an abrasive paste.	Pour ½ cup soda down slow drain, followed by ½ cup vinegar. Then follow with Lemon oil for fresh scent.
Washing Soda (Sodium carbonate decahydrate) or (Soda Ash)	A mineral-based washing soda. Excellent grease and stain remover. Water softener. Mineral de-scaler.	Citrus essential oils can be added to washing soda to enhance any cleaning job.
Club Soda	Carbon dioxide aids in removal of the most difficult laundry stains: blood, wine, coffee, chocolate, tomatoes, etc.	Citrus essential oils can be added to Club Soda to enhance cleaning job.
Diatomaceous Earth (DE) Food Grade	Natural silica-based abrasive. Wear a mask, if used as a dry powder. Sprinkle around doorways and windows to deter insect pests. May be mixed with water or vinegar to form an abrasive paste. Excellent for cleaning porcelain surfaces.	Citrus essential oils can be added to DE/water-based paste to enhance the cleaning process. Thieves oil is excellent with DE in paste form for cleaning toilets and other porcelain surfaces.
Hydrogen Peroxide	An excellent whitening/oxidizing agent with 3% solution. Oxidizes bacteria, making it antimicrobial. Alternative to bleach. Deters molds and mildews.	1/3 Hydrogen Peroxide to 2/3 water in a 32-oz bottle with a capful of Thieves Cleaner make a powerful all-purpose cleaner. Stain remover.
SALT or NaCl (Sodium Chloride)	Cleans, disinfects, deodorizes Neutral in pH, saline (water with salt) excellent antimicrobial solution for rags and sponges.	Lemon oil with salt is a rust remover.
VINEGAR or Acetic Acid (all forms)	Slightly acidic makes it a natural antimicrobial. Denatures protein residues on surfaces, such as glass and mirrors.	Citrus oils can be added to vinegar to enhance its cleaning properties.
Vegetable-based Oils (fractionated coconut, olive, avocado, sweet almond, jojoba)	Excellent carrier oils for DIY products. Use in spray bottle to polish furniture, stainless steel, natural stone, etc. Can be used to prevent dryness of leather.	Lemon oil with a vegetable-based carrier is excellent for removing sticky gum residues.
Neutral Spirits (Alcohols) Vodka	Highly concentrated, food-grade alcohols. Odor eliminators. Streak-free shine when used on glass. Polishes surfaces. Use vodka in place of ammonia	Purification and geranium oils in water and vodka base deters insect pests.
Castile Soap	Olive Oil base with KOH to denature proteins.	Soap-base with essential oils added for DIY soap products; foaming hand soap.

*These materials are suggested for use as common DIY ingredients. Often you have them in your kitchen, laundry room, even bathroom. You are encouraged to use the Young Living Product guide in support of the essential oils required in the forthcoming recipes. Have fun.

MOMS/WOMEN

"A mother's arms are made of tenderness, and children sleep soundly in them."
—Victor Hugo

"As we make the move out of the bathroom's medicine cabinet to its vanity, we begin to encounter those products containing phthalates and parabens, the endocrine disruptors. Bathrooms are home to a veritable chemicopia of personal care products." (Thompson).

FACT: On average, women use twice as many personal care products as men, applying far more chemicals to their bodies. Some of these chemicals are completely harmless, others are endocrine disruptors, carcinogens and neurotoxins, most of which have not been independently reviewed for safety before hitting store shelves (Guardian).

FACT: Your skin is your body's largest organ. Though protective, it also is permeable, so chemicals placed on the skin are absorbed through the skin. Once toxins enter the bloodstream, they potentially accumulate over time, as we cannot metabolize them fast enough or we cannot metabolize them at all.

Let's simplify your routine by making your own products.

For example, many lotions, potions, and hair care product routines can be eliminated with the use of coconut oil combined with high quality essential oils.

"Anything that goes on your body should be safe enough to go in your body."
-D. Gary Young, Young Living Founder & CEO

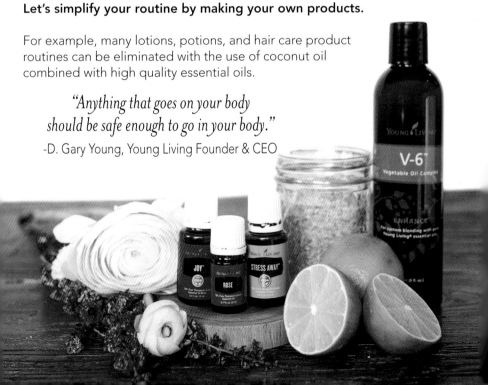

DIY PERSONAL CARE RECIPES

Wake me up Before WE Go-Go Morning Spritzer

- 1 cup sparkling water
- Juice of one lemon
- 2 drops Peppermint oil
- 1 drop Rosemary oil

Mix all ingredients together. Use after cleansing bath or shower. OR use while still in bath or shower sponging over body from head to toe. Rinse off with warm water and towel dry. This recipe can also be put into a spritzer bottle and spritz on your way to work.

Basic Essential Oil Shower Gel

- ½ cup Castile (unscented) soap
- 1 tsp sweet almond oil
- 4 drops essential oil (your choice)
- Makes 4 oz. Store in a 4 oz dispensable bottle

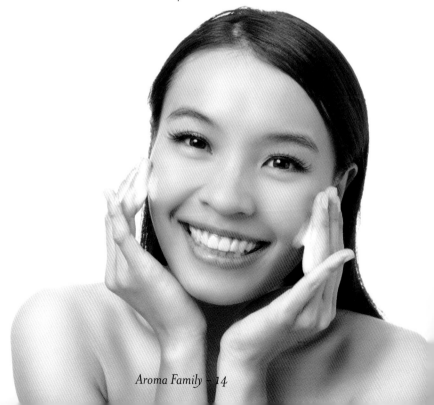

GIRL TALK

For the Girls: Breast Health Oil Rub

- 3 drops Cypress
- 3 drops Frankincense
- Optional: 1 drop Sandalwood

Mix together in 1 tsp V-6 or a favorite skin oil. Apply to armpits and around breasts before bedtime one week per month.

Down There Care: Vaginal Fresh Wash

- 2 drops Melrose
- 1 drop Thyme

Mix the essential oils into the saline water of a douche kit. Douche with the solution in the shower. Use as needed.

ALTERNATIVE: Mix oils with ClaraDerm instead of water in a bowl. Soak a tampon and insert. Can be left in for a couple hours.

That Time of the Month

- 10 drops Geranium
- 10 drops Clary Sage
- 10 drops Bergamot

Massage on abdomen, hops, and lower back OR place 5-10 drops into a warm bath.

Go With the Flow

- 10 drops Dragon Time
- 4 drops Basil
- 2 drops Geranium

Mix oils together in 1 tbsp of your favorite skin oil. Rub on lower back and abdomen. Best when started two days before anticipated period day through the second day of your cycle. One can apply hot compress over lower abdomen or across lower back for added comfort.

For the Bum

(Have you been sitting too long and the rectum is uncomfortable?)
- 1 drop Basil
- ½ tsp olive oil

Dab directly on the rectum.

Love Potion

- 6 drops Ylang Ylang
- 3 drops Patchouli
- 3 drops Joy
- 2 drops Sandalwood
- 2 drops Balsam fir
- 1 drop Cedarwood
- ½ oz V-6 carrier oil

Mix together and put into a small roller ball. Place on your night stand or place in your purse and used as cologne.

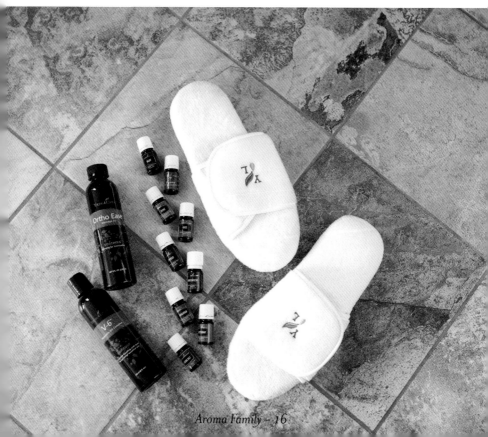

NATURAL BEAUTY SECRETS

Amped Up Working Girl Hair Detangler

- ½ cup Young Living Conditioner
- 1 and 1/8 cup warm distilled water
- 3 drops Cedarwood essential oil
- 3 drops Frankincense essential oil

Mix ingredients together and add to a 16-oz spray bottle. Spritz a couple of times into dry or damp hair and comb through to tame your mane.

On the Go Dry Shampoo

- ¼ cup cornstarch
- 1 tablespoon baking soda
- 2 drops Cedarwood
- 2 drops Rosemary
- 1 drop Tea Tree (*Melaleuca alternifolia*)
- OPTIONAL for those with dark hair: 2 tablespoons unsweetened cocoa powder.

Mix all ingredients. Shake a small amount into your hair and massage the powder into your roots. After a few minutes, comb through your hair for soft, refreshed locks.

Be Good to Your Footsies

- Carrier oil, such as Young Living's V-6 oil
- Lavender or *Eucalyptus globulus* essential oils

At the end of a long day on your feet, add 1 teaspoon of carrier oil to cupped hand and add two drops of lavender or *Eucalyptus globulus*. Massage and rub into feet.

DIY BATH SCRUBS

Blend together 1/3 cup each (equal parts) of the following:
* 1/3 cup Epsom Salts (muscle relaxant, detoxifier)
* 1/3 cup Celtic Salts (mineral-rich)
* 1/3 cup Baking Soda (skin softener)
* 5 – 10 drops favorite essential oil or oil blend

Add 5 – 10 drops of your favorite essential oil to the blend and then add to warm bath water or apply to your body as a "Salt Glow." Rub prior to bath. Adding a spoonful of a favorite carrier oil to the "Salt Glow" leaves the skin feeling soft and silky. Essential oil suggestions include, Patchouli, Sandalwood, or Lavender oils.

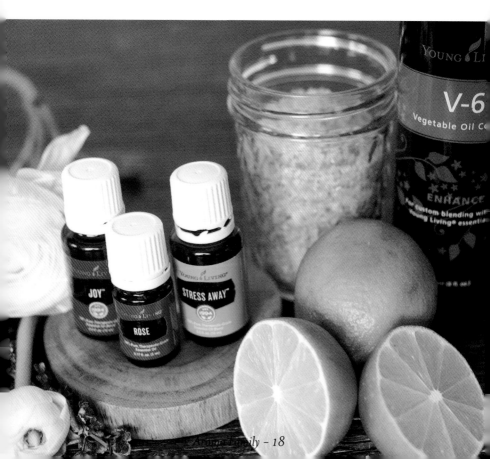

From the Fields Salt Scrub

- 10 drops Lavender oil
- 10 drops Rosemary oil
- 2 cups organic coconut oil
- 1 cup salt (Pink Himalayan)
- Small Mason jars with lids

In a small bowl, mix the coconut oil and salt together. Add the essential oils and continue to stir together. When blended, store in wide-mouth jars with tight-fitting lids. At shower or bath time, scoop the scrub with two fingers and gently rub over skin, then rinse. After use, rinse shower stall floor well with hot water, as floor may be slippery.

Skin So Soft Body Scrub

- ½ cup coconut oil
- 1 cup granulated sugar (fine)
- 10 drops Lavender oil
- 10 drops Sandalwood oil

Combine ½ cup coconut oil with 1 cup fine, granulated sugar. Mix together, then add and mix in essential oils to form a paste. Store in a clean, capped glass jar. Use in the shower.

Mojito Body Scrub

- 3 tablespoons sugar
- 1 tablespoon Grapeseed oil
- 1 tablespoon Jojoba oil
- 8 drops Lime essential oil
- 4 drops Peppermint essential oil

In a small bowl, mix oils and sugar. In shower or bath, apply the sugar scrub in gentle circular motions. Rinse. Single use recipe. If recipe is doubled, then store in a glass container in a dark, cool location.

YOUR BEST SKIN CARE ROUTINE

The following essential oils are excellent skin-supportive oils: Frankincense, Myrrh, Sandalwood, Lavender, Rose, Geranium, Ylang Ylang, Patchouli, Helichrysum, and others.

STEP 1: SKIN CARE CLEANSE

FACIAL STEAM:
- Disperse 3 or 5 drops of Bergamot and Frankincense in a teaspoon of milk or honey and mix into a pint of hot water.
- Pour this heated mixture into a stainless steel mixing bowl and place your face over the rising steam.
- Cover your head with a towel to catch the steam onto your face, breath in and relax, enjoying this facial steam until the water cools. Oils may also be used in a facial steamer.

NOTE to user: essential oils are not water soluble. The steam acts as a dispersant for the oil droplets resting on top of the water's surface. Oils added to a facial steamer or even bath water may cause the oils to penetrate the skin more quickly, causing irritation to sensitive or damaged skin (blemishes, sores, or rash). Use with care.

FACIAL OIL BLEND:
- 10 drops of an essential oil (your choice)
- 1 oz of a carrier oil (avocado, coconut, almond, V-6)
- Small amber, bottle

Mix essential oil with carrier oil in a small, capped, dispensing bottle (amber in color). Dispense a small amount to cupped hand. Rub between two hands and gently apply to face.

SKIN BRUSHING: Invigorate skin and stimulate the body's lymphatic system with this recipe.

- Apply 1 drop of a skin invigorating oil, such as lavender, sandalwood, or geranium to one tablespoon of honey and apply mixture to a natural bristle skin brush.
- Brush your skin with the mixture using gently, upward toward the heart, brush strokes.
- Brush from the fingers up to the shoulders, from the toes up to the neck; include the front and the back sides of the body as you breathe deeply. Your skin will feel tingly and refreshed.

NOTE to user: Always work from the extremities of the body upward toward the heart. Omit the face and neck from this cleansing ritual. It is especially effective in the shower.

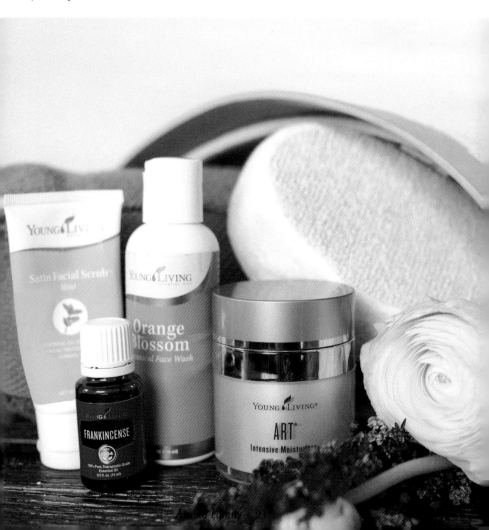

STEP 2: EXFOLIATE

Exfoliating Lip Scrub

- 1 teaspoon brown sugar
- 1 teaspoon honey
- 1 teaspoon coconut oil
- 1 to 2 drops of an essential oil (your choice) in a bowl

Combine ingredients. Mix with a coffee stirrer until a paste forms. To use, gently rub onto lips in a circular motion, rinse or wipe off. Store in an airtight container. Citrus oils are not suggested for this scrub.

Energizing Facial Scrub

- 1 cup rolled oats
- 1/3 cup cornmeal
- 1/3 cup dried peppermint herb
- 4 oz spray bottle
- 1 tsp. vegetable glycerin
- 4 oz distilled water
- 5 drops Peppermint
- 5 drops Sandalwood

Using a coffee grinder, pour in rolled oats, cornmeal, and dried peppermint herb. Grind the mixture to a fine powder. Store in a tightly sealed container for up to 3 months. Un-cap the spray bottle and add 4 oz of distilled water and 1 tsp. of glycerin. Then add the Peppermint and Sandalwood oils.

To use as a scrub, spray open hand with liquid mixture and then add one tablespoon of ground mixture into the liquid of cupped hand. Spray the top of the ground mixture to wet it. Now, rub your hands together to make a paste and apply to face. Scrub. Then rinse with warm water and pat dry with a towel.

Morning Mint Face Scrub

- 5 drops Peppermint oil
- 1 drop Sandalwood oil
- 1 drop Geranium oil
- 1 drop Lavender oil
- 1 drop Frankincense oil
- ¼ cup Greek yogurt
- ¼ cup fine-grained cornmeal

Mix together and add to a capped container. To use, scoop two fingers into mixture and apply to face. Gently scrub, then rinse with warm water. Refrigerate any unused mint scrub.

Sweet Lavender Facial Scrub

- 1 tsp lavender buds
- 1 tablespoon organic sugar
- 1 oz Jojoba oil
- 10 drops Lavender oil
- 2 oz Mason jar with lid

Mix dry ingredients together in a 2 oz jar. Then add the Jojoba oil and the lavender oil to the mix. Scoop enough to apply to the face. Scrub, rinse, and enjoy.

STEP 3: TONE

Sweet Lavender Toner

- ½ cup Filtered water
- ½ cup Raw Apple Cider Vinegar
- 5 drops Sandalwood essential oil
- 5 drops Frankincense essential oil
- ALTERNATIVE Oils: Palo Santo and Lavender

Directions: Mix vinegar and filtered water. Add a few drops of essential oils to the mixture. Use a glass bottle and store at room temperature.

Note: Witch hazel can be substituted for vinegar. Aloe and/or green tea can be added.

Note: Lavender, Melissa, Lemon can be substituted.

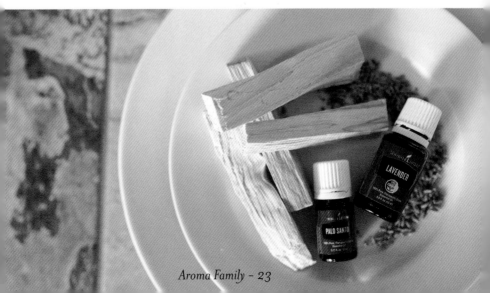

STEP 4: RESTORE

Skin Serum Rejuvenator

After a shower, combine
- 1 to 3 drops of Frankincense and/or Rose
- 1 to 3 drops of Geranium and/or Patchouli
- 1 oz carrier oil (avocado, coconut, almond, V-6).

Rub the body briskly all over and allow the skin to air dry.

Alternative: 1 to 3 drops of each Frankincense, Rose and Patchouli combined with V-6.

Note: Can be mixed in a glass bottle with eyedropper top OR in larger quantities. It may seem like an investment, but you will see that each recipe comes to pennies per application.

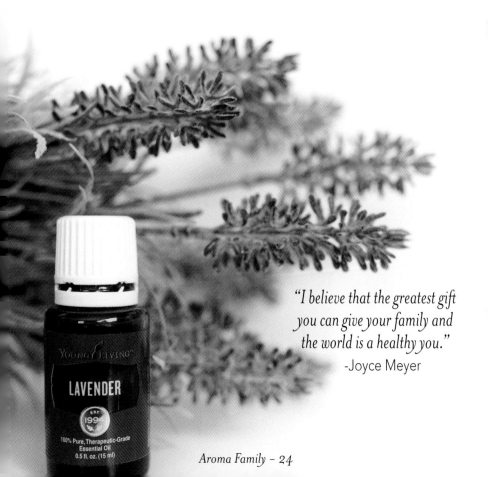

"I believe that the greatest gift you can give your family and the world is a healthy you."
-Joyce Meyer

STEP 5: MOISTURIZE

*Avocado: Avocado is an excellent ingredient for DIY face masks for dry skin.
*Coconut: A go-to ingredient in many DIY personal care products.

Lavender & Rosewater Moisturizer

- 2 tablespoons Rosewater (1 drop Rose essential oil with1/2 cup water)
- 5 drops Lavender oil
- 1 tablespoon coconut oil
- 1 tablespoon avocado oil
- ¼ tsp vegetable glycerin
- Optional: 5 drops Frankincense oil (skin supportive)

Mix all ingredients and add to a cosmetic bottle. Place two or three drops of mixture into a cupped hand, rub both hands together, and apply to face. Mixture will absorb into the skin readily.

Silky Whipped Body Butter

- 1 cup coconut oil
- 1 tablespoon avocado oil
- 5 drops Peppermint oil
- 5 drops Rosemary oil
- 5 drops Lemon oil
- 5 drops *Eucalyptus radiata* oil
- Other oils may be substituted as to your preference.
- V-6 may be substituted for the coconut and avocado oil

Place coconut oil and avocado oil in a chilled mixing bowl. Using a stand or hand mixer, whip the two oils together. Then slowly add in the various essential oils. Continue to whip until creamy and wisp-like peaks are produced. Place into 2- to 4-oz Mason jars with lids. Store in cool location.

STEP 6: REFINE

Hydrating Facial Masque

- 2 to 3 drops of an essential oil (your choice)
- 2 tablespoons of moistened clay, honey, mashed avocado, or egg white
- Small mixing bowl

Apply a thin layer of the mask to your face, and let it sit for 10 to 15 minutes. Then rinse with warm water.

DADS/MEN

*"Dads are most ordinary men turned by love
into heroes, adventurers, story-tellers,
and singers of song."*
—Pam Brown

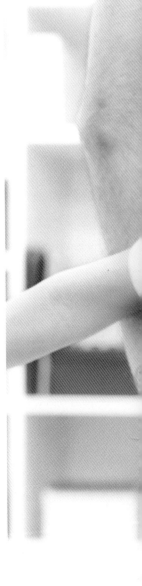

Man Soak

- 1 cup Epsom Salts
- 10 drops essential oil (your choice)
  Suggestions: Idaho Blue Spruce, Shutran,
  Northern Lights Black Spruce

Mix well and store in an airtight jar. To use, pour ½ of mixture into warm bath water.

Hand Purifier

- ¼ cup Aloe Vera gel
- ½ teaspoon glycerin
- 1 tablespoon Vodka
- 10 drops Cinnamon Bark oil
- 10 drops Tea Tree oil
*(Other oil choices depending on preference:
Lemongrass, Purification, Peppermint, Lavender,
Melaleuca alternifolia)*

Mix together in a bowl and disperse into a lotion bottle. Rub into hands several times a day.

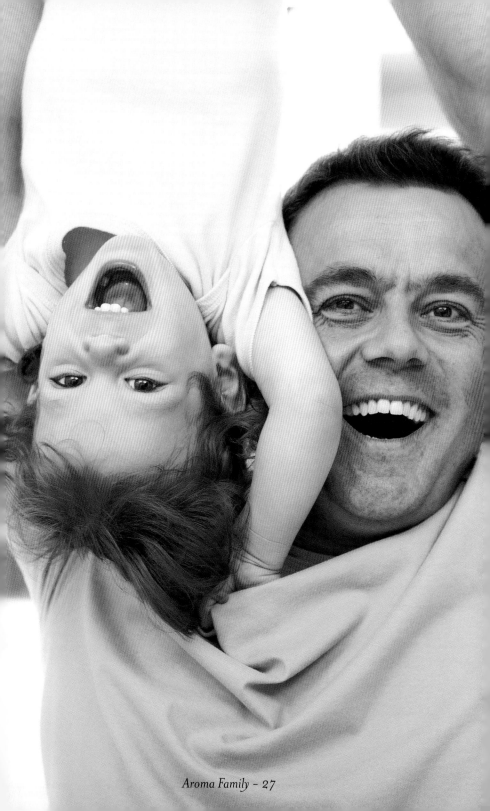

Essential Oils Blend for MTL (Muscles-tendons-ligaments)

- Empty 15 ml oil bottle (remove dropper top)
- 25 drops Wintergreen
- 20 drops Peppermint
- 15 drops Copaiba
- 10 drops Frankincense
- 10 drops Lemongrass
- 5 drops Oregano
- 5 drops Ginger
- 5 drops Cypress

Remove dropper top from an empty 15 ml amber colored oil bottle. Add all of the oils listed with the amounts listed. Add dropper top. Cap, shake, and use on joints, ligaments, and tendons. Rub in 4-5 drops morning, noon, and night, prior to bedtime.

MTL Bath (Muscles-tendons-ligaments)

- 5 drops Peppermint oil (added to baking soda)
- 10 drops Wintergreen oil (added to baking soda)
- ½ Epsom Salt (muscle relaxant, detoxifier)
- ½ cup Baking Soda
  (skin softener and dispersing agent for oils)

In a mixing cup add baking soda and drop Peppermint and Wintergreen oils onto the soda. Mix together with a spoon or wooden skewer. Fill tub with warm water and add baking soda and Epsom Salt to the water, mixing with hand. This is an excellent bath to ease sore, tired, achy muscles of legs, shoulders, and back.

MTL Rub (Muscles-tendons-ligaments)

- 16 oz coconut oil
- 4 oz beeswax pastilles or beeswax shavings
- 1 teaspoon cayenne pepper
- 15 drops Wintergreen oil
- 10 drops Cypress oil
- 10 drops Lemongrass oil
- 10 drops *Eucalyptus radiata* oil
- 10 drops Peppermint oil

Using a double boiler, add coconut oil and beeswax and heat over low heat until the beeswax melts. Once melted, pull pan from heat and add cayenne pepper and all the oil additions. Whisk together. Use a funnel and pour into small Mason jars or small metal screw top containers. Cayenne pepper may disperse to the bottom. Rub should be soft enough to access the pepper residue resting on the bottom. Gently rub into compromised MTL areas.

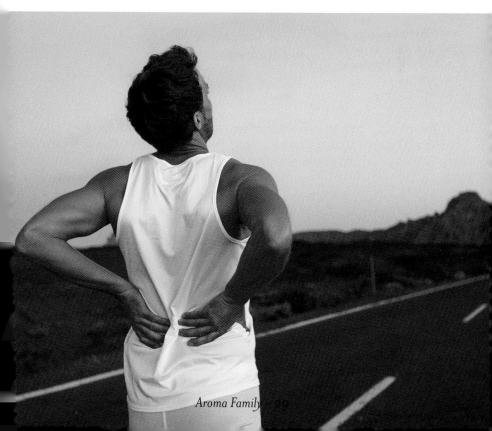

Man Up Deodorant

- ½ coconut oil (melted)
- ¼ cup cornstarch or arrowroot powder for more sensitive skin
- ¼ cup baking soda (pH control)
- 10 drops Patchouli
- 10 drops Cedarwood
- 10 drops Sandalwood
- 10 drops Frankincense
- 10 drops Myrrh
- 10 drops Clove

Mix all ingredients to a paste. Consistency may be adjusted with more or less dry ingredient additions. Add paste to a deodorant container and refrigerate. Keep cool to maintain solid nature.

Man Up Cologne

- Small spray or spritz bottle
- 3 oz water
- 1 tablespoon Vodka
- 10 drops Patchouli
- 10 drops Cedarwood
- 10 drops Sandalwood
- 10 drops Frankincense
- 10 drops Clove
- 10 drops Vetiver

Add 3 oz of water to a small bottle with spray or spritz screw-top attachment. Add 1 tablespoon of vodka. Then add all of the oils listed with the amounts listed. Use as an aftershave and spray at the neck.

Citrus Mint Foot Scrub

- 10 drops Peppermint oil
- 10 drops Lime oil
- 10 drops Orange oil
- 2 oz avocado oil
- 2 cups Epsom Salt
- Glass mixing bowl
- Plastic basin or foot tub
- Towel for drying feet after use

Mix salts, essential oils, carrier oil, in a mixing bowl. Add warm water to foot basin/tub. Scoop out scrub and apply to feet, gently massaging and rubbing into the skin. Concentrate on heels and other calloused areas. Rinse and dry with a towel.

Smooth Talker Body Salve

- Double bowler
- 8 oz. sweet almond oil
- ¼ cup grated beeswax or beeswax pastilles
- 10 drops Sandalwood oil
- 20 drops essential oil of choice
  (Sacred Mountain, Northern Lights Black Spruce, Idaho Balsam, Idaho Blue Spruce, Abundance)
- 10 drops vitamin E

Using a double boiler over low heat, add the almond oil and the beeswax. Heat until the beeswax has melted. Remove from heat and add Sandalwood, oil of choice, and vitamin E. Pour into Mason jar or capped containers and allow mixture to solidify before use. Apply to areas of dry, chapped skin.

Wake Me up Shower Disks

- Mini-muffin tin with paper liners
- Large glass mixing bowl
- 3 cups baking soda
- 1 cup water
- 20 drops Peppermint oil
- 20 drops *Eucalyptus radiata* oil
- 20 drops Tea Tree (*Melaleuca alternifolia*) oil

In a bowl, mix soda and water into a thick paste. Add the essential oils. Stir and spoon into paper liners of mini-muffin tin. Let sit for 1-2 days to allow dehydration of water. Pop out disks from liners and place on the shower stall floor. Take shower and reap the aromatic benefits.

Soothing Hand Cream

- 1 tablespoon Sulfurzyme
- 1 cup coconut oil
- 10 drops Geranium oil
- 10 drops Myrrh Oil
- 10 drops Frankincense oil
- 10 drops Sandalwood oil

Mix all ingredients well in a bowl using a spoon. Dispense into a small Mason jar. Use especially on dry, chapped, hands.

Man Hands Moisturizing Salve

- Using a double boiler, gently heat 8 oz of sweet almond or avocado oil over low heat (both oils can be used together…4 oz of each).
- Add 2 oz of grated beeswax or beeswax pellets and stir until melted (beeswax controls viscosity)
- Remove from heat and add one mL of vitamin E (antioxidant)
- Add 10 drops Sandalwood oil
- Add 10 drops Tea Tree (*Melaleuca alternifolia*) oil
- Add 15 drops Rosemary Oil
- Add 5 drops Lemon Oil

Pour into salve containers with screw-top lids. Cool to allow solidification and store in a cool place to maintain solid-nature.

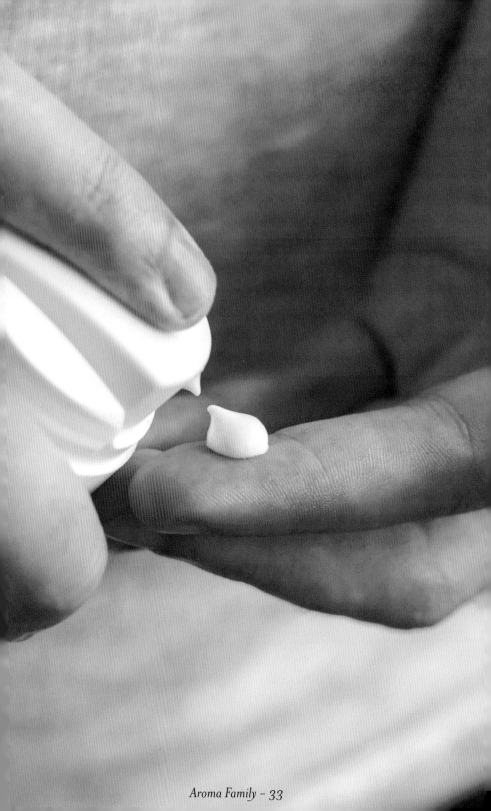

Breathe Easy

- Fill face-sized glass bowl with steaming hot water.
- Add 4 – 8 drops of respiratory assistive oils, such as Lemon, Peppermint, R.C. blend, *Eucalyptus radiata* or *Eucalyptus globulus* oils.
- Keep eyes closed.
- Place face above bowl and drape a towel over head to catch the rising vapors.
- Inhale water until it cools, no longer releasing vapors.
- Repeat as needed several times during the day to relieve sinus congestion, sore throat, cough and cold symptoms.

Bug Bars

(for hunting, camping or play - makes 12 small bars)
- 3 oz beeswax pastilles
- 1.5 cups cocoa butter
- 2 oz sweet Almond oil
- 1 tsp Vodka
- 4 drops vitamin E (antioxidant)
- 3 drops *Eucalyptus radiata* oil
- 3 drops Cedarwood oil
- 3 drops Lemongrass oil
- 3 drops Sandalwood oil
- 3 drops Geranium oil
- Mini-muffin tin lined with paper liners.
  Spray liners with avocado or coconut cooking spray.

Using a double boiler, in the top pan add beeswax, cocoa butter, and almond oil. Heat on low until all have liquefied. Remove from heat and stir in vodka, vitamin E, and the essential oils. Pour liquid into pre-sprayed paper liners in a mini-muffin tray. Allow the bars to cool and solidify. Bars can stay in paper liners or they may be removed. Rub over skin.

On the Go Car Diffuser

- Pom-poms
- Essential oils (your choice)
- Clips (small magnet clips or wooden clothes pins)

Place several drops of an essential oil (your choice) onto pom-pom. Clip pom-pom to car vent with a magnet clip or wooden clothes pin and allow the air flow of the car vent to disperse the essential oil.

"My father gave me the greatest gift anyone could give another person: he believed in me."
—Jim Valvano

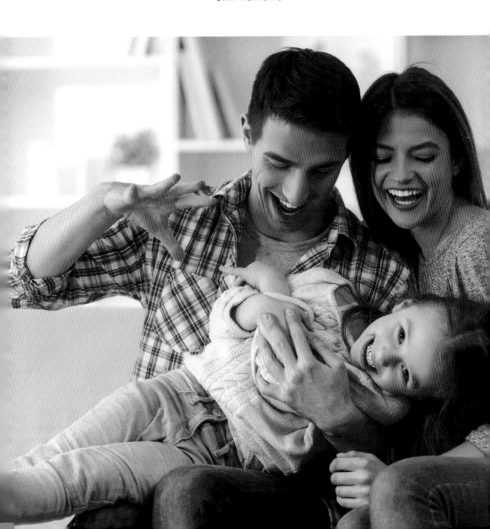

CHILDREN

"Obviously you would give your life for your children, or give them the last biscuit on the plate. But to me, the trick in life is to take that sense of generosity between kin, make it apply to the extended family, to your neighbor, your village, and beyond."
-Tom Stoppard

The following essential oils are supportive for children:
Jasmine, Lemongrass, Ylang Ylang, Lavender, Chamomile, Frankincense, Sandalwood, Cedarwood, Helichrysum, the Citrus Oils, Bergamot, (Caution: the Citrus Oils and Bergamot are photosensitive oils)

HOMEWORK HAVEN:
Prior to homework, diffuse any of the following enlightening scents: Rosemary, Lemon, Sage, Peppermint, *Eucalyptus globulus.*

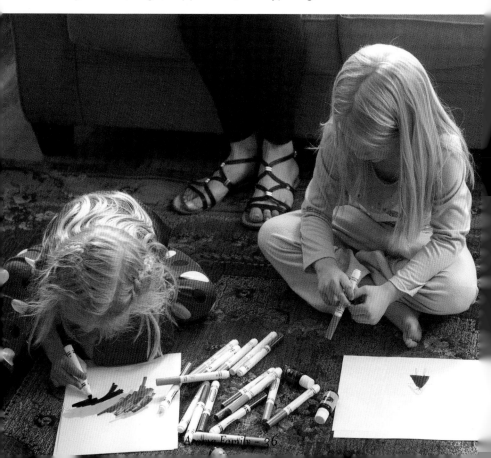

DIY PERSONAL CARE

Chill Pill Back Rub

Mix 10 drops Lavender, 4 drops Roman Chamomile, 10 drops Petitgrain, 1 drop Myrtle in small glass sample bottle. Shake. Then dilute 3 drops of this mixture in 1 tsp of your favorite skin oil and rub over the both temples and middle forehead. Be sure to avoid the eye area.

Dry Scalp Oil Rub

- 1 oz jojoba oil
- 15 drops Carrot Seed oil

Use a small amount and rub into the scalp. This mix may stain your pillow case so use old sheets. In the morning, use the gentlest shampoo you can find. KidScents Shampoo is recommended.

To 4 oz of shampoo add:
- 10 drops Tea Tree
- 10 drops Manuka
- 5 drops Myrtle

Open the Airways

- 10 drops Ravintsara
- 10 drops Thyme
- 5 drops *Eucalyptus radiata*
- 1 tsp almond oil or other skin oil

Add a small amount to hands. Rub hands together and apply to child's chest and back.

Breathe Better Bars

- ½ cup sweet almond oil
- 2 tablespoons of beeswax pastilles
- 5 drops *Eucalyptus radiata*
- 1 drop Rosemary
- 2 drops Chamomile

In a double boiler, add beeswax pastilles to sweet almond oil. Using low heat, melt beeswax into almond oil. Once pastilles are melted, remove from heat. Stir in *Eucalyptus radiata*, Rosemary, and Chamomile oil additions.

Bath Fun & Bubbles

- 8 oz Foaming Hand Soap Dispenser
- 6 oz distilled water
- 1 tsp fractionated coconut oil
- 3 tablespoons Castile Soap
- 10 drops essential oil (Lavender, Orange, Gentle Baby)

Stir with a spoon to slowly blend all ingredients in a small bowl. Use a funnel to pour into a soap dispenser. Add pump and use.

Owie Boo-Boo Spray

- 8 oz spray bottle
- 8 oz distilled water
- 8 drops Lavender essential oil
- 4 drops Tea Tree (*Melaleuca alternifolia*) essential oil
- 2 drops Chamomile
- 2 drops Cypress
- 1 drop Sandalwood

Un-cap bottle and fill to the neck with distilled water. Add all essential oil ingredients. Shake thoroughly before use. Spray on offended area several times a day. Convenient to carry in pocket or backpack.

The Great Outdoors Spray

- Fill an 8-oz spray bottle with 4 ounces of distilled water.
- Add 4-oz of Witch Hazel
- Add 10 drops each of the following essential oils: Thieves, Purification, Peppermint

Shake well and spray on skin often.

Sun Soothed Lips

- 1 tablespoon beeswax pastilles
- 1 tablespoon Shea butter
- 2 tablespoons sweet almond oil
- 1 tablespoon coconut oil
- 15 drops Lavender essential oil
- 5 drops Sandalwood oil
- 2-3 drops vitamin E (antioxidant)

Using a double boiler, add beeswax, Shea butter, almond oil, and coconut oil to the top pan. Heat on low until the beeswax melts completely. Remove from heat and add vitamin E and essential oil additions. Pour into small, screw-top lid, metal containers. Allow mixture to cool and solidify. Best if stored in cool area.

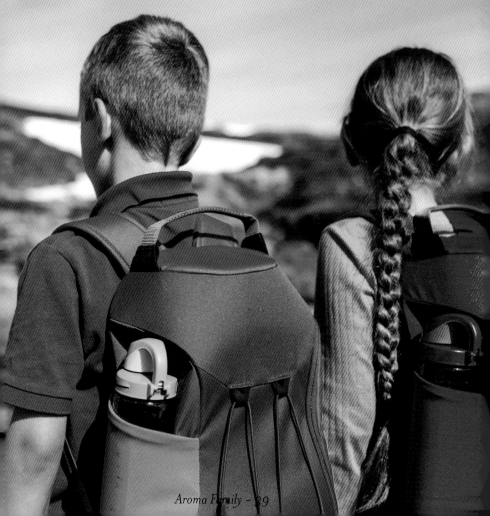

Don't Bug Me Spray

- One cup of vodka or witch hazel
- 40 drops Geranium oil
- 30 drops Lemongrass
- 20 drops *Eucalyptus radiata*

Add to a spray bottle and shake before each use. Use often.

Before going outside, mix 1 tablespoon of olive oil with 1 drop Geranium oil and 1 drop Lemongrass oil and wipe around ankles, wrists, and neck. After day outdoors, shower and wash head thoroughly. Afterwards, perform a thorough check of child's hair and body.

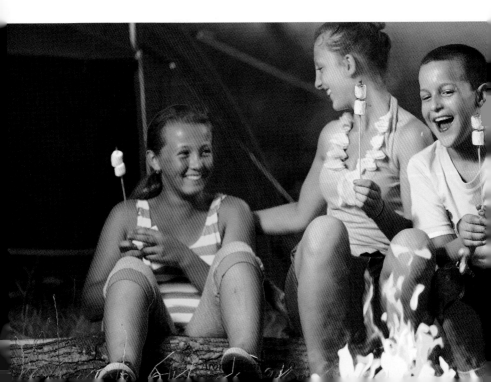

Fun in the Sun Spray

- ½ sweet almond oil
- ¼ cup coconut oil (natural SPF 4)
- ¼ beeswax pastilles or shaved from bar
- 2 tablespoons Zinc Oxide (Take care NOT to inhale powder)
- 2 tablespoons Shea Butter (natural SPF 4)
- 20-30 drops of Carrot Seed Oil (Carotenoid pigments, excellent for sun protection)
- 10 drops Myrrh Oil (skin supportive)
- 10 – 20 drops essential oil(s), your choice for added scent (Do not choose photoactive oils, such as Bergamot, or any of the citrus oils)
- Optional: 1 tsp vitamin E (excellent antioxidant for skin health)

Use a double boiler and in the top place the almond oil, coconut oil, Shea butter, and beeswax. Heat on low until the beeswax has melted into the oil mixture. Remove from heat and quickly stir in all of the essential oil additions, along with the vitamin E. Then stir in the Zinc Oxide and pour into a storage container, such as a pint-sized Mason jar. Store in a cool, dry location or in the refrigerator. The recipe has an SPF of approximately 15; however SPF can be increased with the addition of more Zinc Oxide. The texture and hardness of the sunscreen is determined by the amount of beeswax added to the recipe. Adjustments can be made with the beeswax ingredient to achieve the proper consistency for you.

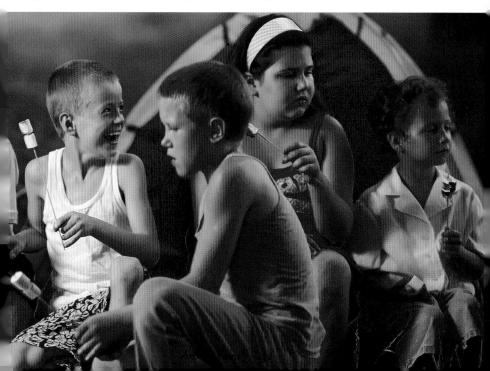

Sweet Dreams Bedtime Cream

- 1 cup coconut oil
- 2 tablespoons beeswax pastilles
- 5 drops Sandalwood
- 10 drops Lavender
- 4 drops vitamin E (antioxidant)

Add coconut oil and beeswax pellets to the top of a double boiler. Over low heat melt the beeswax pellets into the coconut oil. Pull pan off of heat source and add essential oils and vitamin E. Stir and pour into a small Mason jar. Cool. It will loosely solidify into a cream. Apply to child's feet at night in preparation for sleep. Optional: Pour melted coconut oil and liquefied beeswax into a small, chilled mixing bowl, add oils and then whip with an electric mixer for a BEDTIME WHIP. Spoon into a small Mason jar and store in a cool location.

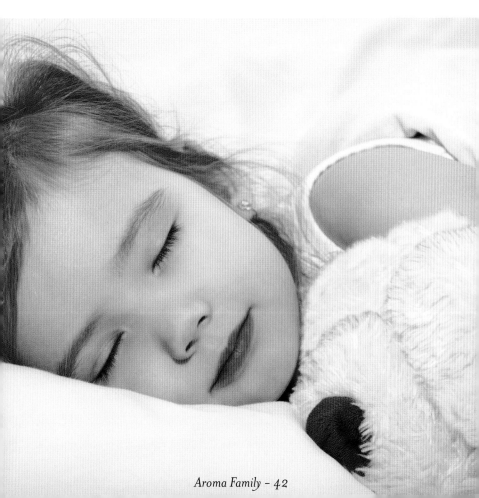

Rise & Shine

- 1 cup coconut oil
- 2 tablespoons beeswax pastilles
- 5 drops Sandalwood
- 10 drops Lemon
- 4 drops vitamin E (antioxidant)

Add coconut oil and beeswax pellets to the top of a double boiler. Over low heat melt the beeswax pellets into the coconut oil. Pull pan off of heat source and add essential oils and vitamin E. Stir and pour into a small Mason jar. Cool. It will loosely solidify into a cream. Apply to child's feet in the morning for a-get-ready-for-your-day experience. Optional: Pour melted coconut oil and liquefied beeswax into a small, chilled mixing bowl, add oils and then whip with an electric mixer for a MORNING WHIP. Spoon into a small Mason jar and store in a cool location.

Twinkle Toes

- 2 tablespoons baking powder
- 5 drops your child's favorite essential oil

Mix together. Spoon a tablespoon of mixture into each shoe and shake shoe to disperse. Leave overnight or longer, then shake out of shoes.

"Give a little love to a child, and you get a great deal back."
-John Ruskin

WHOLE FAMILY COOKING

"A happy family is but an earlier heaven."
-George Bernard Shaw

Citrus Vinaigrette

- ½ cup olive or avocado oil
- 2 cloves garlic, minced
- 1 shallot, minced
- 2 – 3 drops Lime Vitality oil
- 3 – 4 drops Tangerine Vitality oil
- 2 – 3 drops Lemon Vitality oil
- 2 drops Black Pepper Vitality oil
- 1 – 2 tablespoons honey for a sweetening touch
- A dash of salt to taste
- A sprinkle of dried parsley

Add all to a small Mason jar, shake and use on a fresh salad or on a fresh vegetable mix. Can be mixed with cream cheese and sour cream for a refreshing veggie dip.

Store in the refrigerator.

Essential Oil Vinaigrette for Salads or Veggies

- ¾ cup extra virgin olive oil
- ¼ cup vinegar
- 2 drops Vitality Black Pepper oil
- 2 drops Vitality "flavorful" oil (Oregano, Sage, Rosemary, Thyme) or mix any two

Place all in a shake container with top. Always shake, prior to use.

Lemon Dill Sauce for Meat, Veggies or Both

- ½ cup dry white wine
- ½ cup plain Greek yogurt
- 2 cloves garlic, minced
- ½ teaspoon Dijon mustard
- 3 tablespoons unsalted butter, divided
- ½ teaspoon salt
- Pinch cayenne pepper
- 3 drops Young Living Vitality Lemon Oil
- 3 drops Young Living Vitality Dill Oil
- 3 drops Young Living Vitality Black Pepper Oil

1. Add together white wine and minced garlic in a saucepan over medium heat.
2. Bring to a boil and boil for about two minutes.
3. Reduce heat to simmer and whisk in yogurt and Dijon mustard. Continue to simmer as the sauce thickens.
4. Remove from heat and whisk in butter pieces.
5. Finally add essential oils and salt and pepper to taste.

Use as a sauce for grilled meats, vegetables, or both.

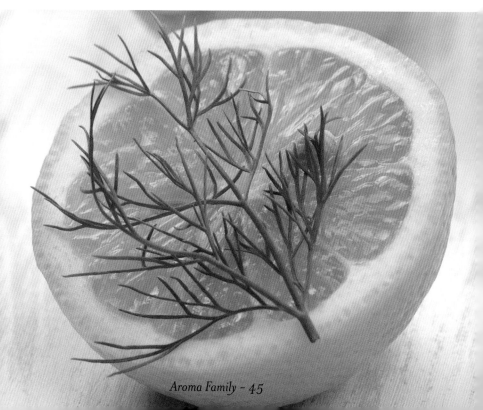

Basic Vinaigrette/Marinade

- 3 tablespoons olive oil (or other oil of your choice)
- 2 tablespoons vinegar (your choice) or 2 tablespoon lemon juice (acid addition)
- Vitality essential oil additions: Oregano, Basil, Thyme, Rosemary, Dill, Ginger, Tarragon, Black Pepper, Sage, Citrus oils (Lemon, Orange, Lime, Grapefruit, Tangerine), Cinnamon Bark, Clove, Nutmeg

Can be used to dress salads, vegetables, or as a meat marinade.

Beef Marinade

- 2/3 cup fresh pineapple juice
- ¼ cup soy sauce
- 2 teaspoons Agave or Honey
- 1 or 2 drops of Vitality Ginger oil
- 1 or 2 drops of Vitality Black Pepper oil
- Cut steak in strips, salt, and place into bowl.
- Prepare marinade with the addition of pineapple juice, soy sauce, Agave or honey, and the Vitality Ginger and Black Pepper oils. Whisk together.
- Pour marinade over beef strips, cover bowl and allow to marinade several hours in the refrigerator.
- Beef strips can be skewered and cooked over a barbecue flame.

Pork Marinade

- ¼ cup of Tart Cherry Juice
- ¼ cup olive oil
- 1 tablespoon Agave or Honey
- 2 drops Vitality Black Pepper oil
- 2 to 3 drops Vitality Sage oil
- Cut pork into strips or if tenderloin cut, then slice into pork medallions, salt, and place into a bowl.
- Prepare marinade with the addition of tart cherry juice, olive oil, agave or honey, Vitality Black Pepper oil and Vitality Sage oil. Whisk together.
- Pour marinade over pork, cover bowl and allow to marinade several hours in the refrigerator.
- Pork strips can be skewered and cooked over a barbecue flame. Pork medallions can also be cooked on a barbecue grill.

Chicken Marinade

- ¼ cup olive oil
- Juice of a whole lemon (remove seeds)
- 1 tablespoon Agave or honey
- 2 drops Vitality Black Pepper oil
- 2 to 3 drops Vitality Tarragon oil
- Cut chicken into "tender-sized" strips, salt, and place into a bowl.
- Prepare marinade with olive oil, lemon juice, agave or honey, Vitality Black Pepper oil, and Vitality Tarragon oil. Whisk together.
- Pour marinade over strips, cover bowl and allow to marinade several hours in the refrigerator.
- Chicken strips can be skewered and cooked over a barbecue flame.

Chicken with Oils Marinade

- ½ cup NingXia Red Juice
- ¼ cup olive oil
- Juice of a whole lemon (remove seeds)
- 2 tablespoons Dijon mustard
- 2 tablespoons of a sweetening agent (honey, agave, or maple syrup)
- 1 drop Vitality Tarragon oil
- 1 drop Vitality Rosemary oil
- 1 drop Vitality Lavender oil
- 1 drop Vitality Black Pepper oil

Whisk all ingredients in a bowl. Salt 4-5 chicken breasts and place into the marinade bowl. Press the chicken breasts into the marinade. Cover and place into refrigerator to marinated overnight. Lightly cover baking pan with olive oil and lay marinated chicken breasts in pan. Pour marinade over the chicken, cover, and bake at 350 F oven for an hour.

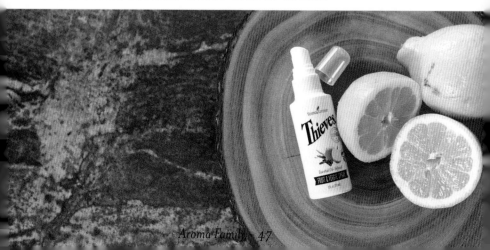

Spiced Butternut Squash Soup

- 3 butternut squash peeled and cut into 6 halves, lengthwise
- 4 cups veggie broth
- 2 drops of Young Living Vitality Nutmeg oil
- 2 drops of Young Living Vitality Cinnamon Bark oil
- 1 drop Young Living Vitality Black Pepper oil
- 6 pats of butter
- 6 garlic cloves
- 2 tablespoons Maple Syrup
- 2 tablespoons light cream
- Salt to taste

Place butternut squash halves onto a cookie sheet pre-oiled with olive oil. Place a garlic clove inside each half and a pat of butter. Cover with foil and bake at 375 F for 1 hour. Allow squash to cool before spooning out squash from rind into a food processor or mixing bowl. Puree with the maple syrup addition and the addition of light cream. Add salt to taste. Add 4 cups of veggie broth to a pot and then stir in pureed squash. Heat on the stove and consistency should be soup-like. Once cooked to desired temperature, stir in essential oil additions. Soup should be smooth in texture and flavorful. It may be garnished with chopped pecans.

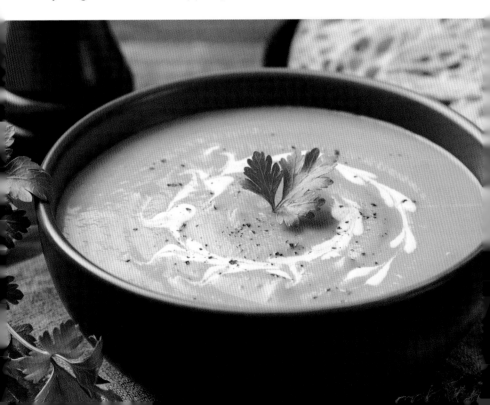

Banana / Zucchini Bread

- 3-4 ripe bananas, smashed
- 1/3 cup melted butter
- ¾ cup granulated sugar
- ¼ cup brown sugar
- 1 egg, beaten
- 1 tsp baking soda
- Pinch of salt
- 1.5 cups of flour (for healthier recipe… use whole wheat flour, etc.)
- Stir in 1-2 cups of shredded zucchini into batter
- Stir in 1 cup of shredded coconut into batter
- Several drops of Vitality essential oils to flavor batter (Experiment with Orange, Cinnamon Bark, Clove, Nutmeg, etc.)

1. Pre-heat oven to 350 F.
2. Using a mixer blend smashed bananas, melted butter, granulated sugar, brown sugar, and egg to a smooth consistency.
3. Add in baking soda, salt, and flour until well mixed.
4. By hand stir in the zucchini and coconut additions.
5. Pre-spray bread loaf pan, add batter, and bake 50 – 60 minutes. Test bread for doneness using a toothpick or wooden skewer; poke and clean means bread is done.

Lavender Lemonade Recipe

- 6 lemons, juiced
- 1 lime, juiced
- ½ cup honey
- 1 drop Lavender Vitality oil
- Ice water, about 10 cups
- Lavender sprigs, optional

1. Combine lemon juice, lime juice, honey in a sauce pan and heat to make a simple syrup.
2. Remove from stove and add 1 drop of Lavender Vitality oil
3. Add syrup to a jug filled with 8 cups of water. Add ice and taste.
4. Stir until well mixed.
5. Garnish with sprigs of lavender.

Raspberry NingXia Sorbet

- 2 cups frozen raspberries
- 2 sliced, frozen bananas
- 2 cups coconut milk
- 100 mL Young Living's NingXia Red Juice
- 1 drop Vitality Peppermint oil
- 1 drop Vitality Lime oil

BLEND all ingredients together. Pour into a glass or metal container & pop into the freezer. Allow to thaw slightly before serving in individual bowls.

Peppermint Brownies with Essential Oils

- 1 15-ounce can of black beans
- 1/3 cup coconut oil
- ¼ cup unsweetened cocoa powder
- 1/8 tsp salt
- 2 tsp vanilla extract
- ½ cup honey
- 3 eggs
- 2 drops Peppermint Vitality oil
- ¼ cup mini-dark chocolate chips

Preheat oven to 350 F. Rinse and drain black beans. Melt coconut until clear. Blend all using hand mixer or food processor until smooth. In a separate bowl, whisk eggs until well beaten. Fold eggs into the chocolate mixture. Add chips and fold. Pour mixture into a greased 8 x 8 baking pan and bake 25-30 minutes. Let cool for 15 minutes and then cut into squares. Allow to cool for an additional 15 minutes and then serve.

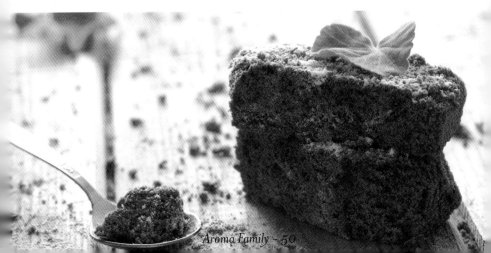

Lemon Crunch Cookies

- Oven temperature 350 F
- ½ cup butter softened
- 1 cup granulated sugar
- ½ tsp almond extract
- Zest of one lemon
- 1 egg
- 15 to 20 drops of Lemon Vitality oil
- ¼ tsp salt
- ¼ tsp baking powder
- 1/8 tsp baking soda
- 1.5 cups flour
- Powdered sugar for coating uncooked cookie ball, prior to baking
- Optional addition: ½ cup white chocolate chips

Cream butter, sugar, almond extract, egg, and Lemon essential oil. Fold in zest addition. Sift in dry ingredients (salt, baking powder, baking soda, and flour) and mix. Dough will be soft/stiff consistency. Spoon dough into hand and form 2-inch ball. Roll ball into powdered sugar and place onto slightly greased cookie sheet. Space cookie balls about 2 inches away from each other on cookie sheet. Cook in 350 degree oven for 10-13 minutes, until cookies are slightly browned.

"You don't choose your family.
They are God's gift to you, as you are to them."
-Desmond Tutu

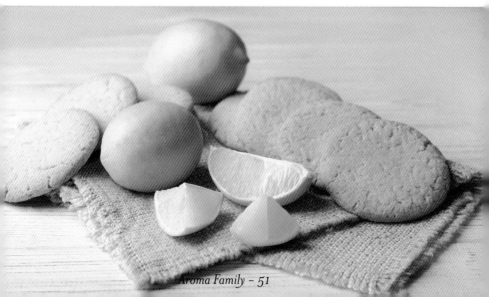

WHAT ABOUT FIDO & KITTY?
HOME CONCERNS (EPA)

HOUSEHOLD SUBSTANCE	CATEGORY INCLUDES	EFFECTS
General Cleaners Even after use of these products, residual vapors can harm pets.	Bleach Drain Cleaners (Lye-base) Ammonia Toilet Bowl Cleaners Chlorine Glycol ethers Formaldehyde	Gastrointestinal ulcers Increases risk of cancer, anemia, liver, kidney damage, skin damage, damage to eyes. Products leave dangerous residues. TOXICITY: varies with exposure
Insecticides (flea & tick) products	Sprays, other application methods	FOLLOW DIRECTIONS Insecticides applied to dogs are not appropriate for cats. Can cause toxicity in cats with vomiting, seizures, and respiratory distress. Yard insecticides never applied to pets.
Oven Cleaners	Ammonia-based	Irritant to Mucous membranes
Window Cleaners	Ammonia-based	Irritant to Mucous membranes
Automatic Dish Detergents	Chlorine	Chlorine is heavier than air and sinks to level of pet. Respiratory irritant.
Tile Scrubs	Chlorine	Chlorine is heavier than air and sinks to level of pet. Respiratory irritant. Dizziness, vomiting. Do not let pets swim in family swimming pool.
Mildew Removers	Chlorine	Chlorine is heavier than air and sinks to level of pet. Respiratory irritant. Dizziness, vomiting Do not let pets swim in family swimming pool.
Toilet Bowl Cleaners	Chlorine	Chlorine is heavier than air and sinks to level of pet. Respiratory irritant. Dizziness, vomiting Do not let pets swim in family swimming pool.
Glass Cleaners Carpet Cleaners Spot Removers	Glycol Ether	Linked to lung damage, anemia, kidney damage in pets and human beings.
Pet Soaps & Pet Shampoos	Formaldehyde	Asthma Carcinogenic (cancer causative)

Our pets are lower to the ground than we are, they breathe at a faster rate, and curiosity can kill more than cats; it can kill dogs too. Only use PET SAFE alternatives, like Young Living's pet line of products.

ANIMALS & PETS

"A family is a unit composed not only of children, but of men, women, an occasional animal, and the common cold."
-Ogden Nash

Animals have extremely sensitive olfactory senses. If oils are used with animals, they must be diluted in very low percentages of less than 1% for use. General uses include: pet wash, grooming spray, fleas and ticks, breath freshener, horseflies, stress and anxiety, pet bedding. Cats are especially sensitive to essential oils, so care must be taken as cats do not metabolize oils as dogs, horses, or humans do. Hydrosols or floral waters are safe for use with cats, though.

Don't Bug Me: Pest Spray

- 2 cups distilled water
- 5 drops Purification
- 1 drops Peppermint
- 1 drops Lavender
- 1 drops Cedarwood
- 1 drops Lemongrass
- 1 tablespoon Vodka

Combine ingredients in a spray bottle. Shake well. Lightly spray and rub into dog's coat. Shake well prior to each use.

Pretty Paws

- 1 cup coconut oil
- 1 cup olive oil
- ¼ cup unrefined Shea butter
- ¼ beeswax pastilles
- 12 drops Lavender essential oil
- 12 drops Frankincense essential oil
- 4 drops Black Pepper oil
- ½ tsp vitamin E

Using a double boiler, mix coconut oil, olive oil, Shea butter, and beeswax. Heat over low heat until beeswax melts. Pull off of heat and stir in essential oils and vitamin E additions. Pour into several small Mason jars and allow to cool. Salve is excellent to use on dog paws prior to walking in snow and ground frost conditions.

You Stink! Odors Be Gone Spray

- 4 oz spray bottle
- 2 oz water
- 1 teaspoon vegetable glycerin
- 3 drops Citronella essential oil
- 2 drops Cedarwood essential oil
- 1 drops *Eucalyptus globulus* essential oil

Mix all ingredients well and pour into a 4 oz plastic spray bottle. Spray dog's coat and rub into fur.

Deep Woods Spray

- One cup of Vodka or Witch Hazel
- 40 drops Geranium oil
- 30 drops Lemongrass
- 20 drops *Eucalyptus radiata*

Add to a spray bottle and shake before each use. Use often.

After day outdoors, do a thorough check of the dog's fur and body.

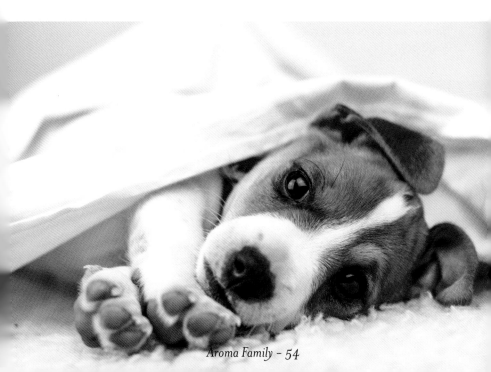

NOT INTO DIY?
TRY SOME OF THESE YOUNG LIVING PRODUCT COMBOS

	VITALITY & PRODUCTIVITY	WOMEN	MEN	EMOTIONS & SLEEP	JOINT HEALTH	ON A TRIP	JOCKS	WEIGHT	DIGEST	STUDENTS	HOME
MultiGreens	√										
Essentialzyme				√		√			√		
Sulfurzyme	√				√						
OmegaGize	√	√	√	√		√				√	
Inner Defense						√					
NingXia Red	√	√	√	√			√	√		√	
Brain Power	√			√							
Mindwise	√									√	
PowerGize			√				√				
BLM					√						
PD 80/20			√								
Thyromin		√									
Life 9									√		
FemiGen		√									
Super C						√					
AgilEase											
Prostate Health			√								
Progessence Plus Serum		√		√							
ImmuPro Tablets				√		√					
Cool Azul Pain Cream					√		√				
Breathe Again						√					
Deep Relief							√				
Digest & Cleanse								√			
Pure Protein							√	√			
Slique Tea						√		√	√		

NOT INTO DIY?
TRY SOME OF THESE YOUNG LIVING PRODUCT COMBOS

	VITALITY & PRODUCTIVITY	WOMEN	MEN	EMOTIONS & SLEEP	JOINT HEALTH	ON A TRIP	JOCKS	WEIGHT	DIGEST	STUDENTS	HOME
Comfortone								√			
Slique Citra Slim								√			
Thieves Cleaner		√	√							√	√
Thieves Tooth		√	√			√				√	√
Thieves Soap		√	√							√	√
Thieves Laundry Detergent		√	√							√	√
Thieves Dishwashing Detergent		√	√							√	√
Thieves Oil						√					√
Peppermint	√					√			√		√
DiGize Oil									√		
Frankincense				√							
Sclar-Essence		√									
Juva Cleanse								√			
Citrus Fresh								√			
Clarity Oil		√	√							√	
Sleep Essence				√							
En-R-Gee Oil										√	
RutaVala				√							
Shutran			√								
Idaho Blue Spruce			√								
Mister			√								
PaloSanto with Lavender				√							
Cedarwood				√							
Lavender				√							

*Use Young Living's Product Guide to aid you in your search for targeted areas.

Here are some categories to guide your search through the product guide:

NOT INTO DIY?

FOR VITALITY
Ningxia Red
OmegaGize3
Essentialzyme-4
MultiGreens
Sulphurzyme Capsules

FOR EMOTIONS
Ningxia Red
OmegaGize3
Essentialzyme-4
Cedarwood
ProGessence Plus
Brain Power
Frankincense

FOR JOINT HEALTH
AgilEase
Sulphurzyme Capsules
BLM
NingXia Red
OmegaGize3
Cool Azul Pain Cream
  Layering combo:
  Copaiba
  Frankincense
  PanAway
  Peppermint
  Alternating combo:
  Idaho Balsam Fir
  Oregano
  Wintergreen
  Peppermint

FOR ON THE GO
TRAVELERS
Slique Tea
ImmuPro tablets
Essentialzyme-4
OmegaGize3
Inner Defense
Thieves Essential Oil Blend
Super C Chewables
Breath-Again roll on
Peppermint

FOR ATHLETES
AgilEase
NingXia Nitro
NingXia Red
PowerGize
Cool Azul Pain Cream
Deep Relief

FOR WOMEN
ProGessence-Plus Serum
FemiGen capsules (or
  EndoGize capsules or
  PD 80/20 capsules)
SclarEssence oil
Thyromin capsules
Thieves Cleaner

FOR MEN
PowerGize
OmegaGize3
PD 80/20
Shutran Beard Cream
Idaho Blue Spruce, Shutran,
  or Mister essential oils

FOR WEIGHT
Pure Protein—Chocolate
  or Vanilla Spice
Juva Cleanse oil
Citrus Fresh oil
Slique Tea
Slique CitraSlim
Comfortone
K & B Tincture
Ningxia Red
Digest & Cleanse
ICP
Slique Product Line

FOR THE HOME
Thieves Household Cleaner
Thieves Toothpaste
Thieves Handsoap
Thieves Laundry
Thieves Dishsoap

FOR DIGESTION
Essentialzyme-4
Life9
Slique Tea
Peppermint
DiGize oil

FOR STUDENTS
MindWise
NignXia Red
OmegaGize3 capsules
Clarity oil
En-R-Gee oil
Brain Power oil
Joy oil
Peppermint

FOR PRODUCTIVITY
MindWise
OmegaGize3
Brain Power
Peppermint

FOR COOKING
Einkorn Flour
Einkorn Pancake Mix
Einkorn Spaghetti, Rotini

FOR ANIMALS
Animal Scents Ointment
Animal Scents Shampoo
Lavender, Copaiba,
Frankincense
Raindrop Technique Kit
Animal Scents Dental
  Pet Chews

FOR ORAL CARE
Thieves Mouthwash
Thieves Dentarome
Toothpaste
Thieves Aromabright
Toothpaste
Thieves Dental Floss
Thieves Lozenges
Thieves Mints
Slique Chewing Gum

FOR SLEEP
Sleep Essence OR
  ImmuPro Capsules
RutaVala OR Palo Santo
combined with Lavender

FOR KIDS
KidScents MightyZymes
KidScents Toothpaste
KidScents Bath Gel
KidScents Shampoo
KidScents Tender Tush
KidScents Lotion

*Depending on what you
are looking for, add your
own categories here and
look through your product
guide and Essential Oil
Desk Reference book to
produce your own lists.*

HOME & FAMILY

"Family makes a house a home."
-Jennifer Hudson

Our homes serve to shelter us, bring us restoration from our busy day and serve as a place of comfort. Yet, so many families unknowingly fill their homes with products that are doing more harm than good. Many consumers are not aware of the harm and so the awareness of hidden toxins in our personal care and cleaning products is an important one. As consumers, we have control over the products we bring into our home environment; it is our responsibility to insure the products are supportive and healthy.

One way to add to our home's protective nature is with the use of essential oils. These gifts from our plant partners possess bioactive compounds nurturing the home environment with their comforting, balancing presence for body, mind, and spirit. Young Living's essential oils with their unquestioned purity provide that presence, whether the oils are diffused, topically applied to the body, or ingested. Our home and our families are the beneficiaries in a Young Living Home. Young Living's oils and its oil-enhanced products including its personal care offerings, the Thieves line of cleaning products, and its nutritional line naturally support our home's living environment, promoting and enhancing it with a cleansing, balancing presence.

Additionally, they provide a calming presence, such as Grounding Essential Oil, diffused at bedtime, acts to relax the mind, uplift our emotions, and rejuvenate our body after an arduous day; so that sleep is more peaceful and restful. With uplifting scents, such as Lemon or Rosemary filling the air, our minds are open to brand new possibilities. A touch of Valor on our collar or at the nape of the neck, reinforces our resolve to make it a success-filled day. The comforting, cleansing presence of essential oils balances our busy lives, so we are better able to address what each day brings. Hence, we are more energized, ready and prepared to be productive and meet those daily responsibilities.

"The family is one of nature's masterpieces."
-George Santayana

WORKS CITED

abcnews.go.com/Health/women-put-on-average-168-chemicals-body-day-consumer/story?id=30615324

Bridges, B. "Fragrance Products Information Network, "N.E.E.D.S. newsletter (1-800-634-1389). Nov. 2—3.

Buckle, Jane. Ph.D. Clinical Aromatherapy. New York. Churchhill Livingstone. 2008.

Burnes, Deborah. "Putting It on Your Skin Does Let It in: What's in Skin Care and How It Affects Your Health." www.huffingtonpost.com/deborah_burnes/skin-care_b_1540929.html.

consumerreports.org/beauty-personal-care/why-is-triclosan-in-toothpaste/

Essential Oils Desk Reference. https://www.discoverlsp.com/all-books/7th-edition-essential-oils-desk-reference.html

ewg.org/enviroblog/2009/03/toxic-personal-care-products-children

www.ewg.org/skindeep/2004/06/15/exposures-add-up-survey-results/

www.kindsoap.com/Ingredients_the_bad.html

Thompson, Athena. Homes that Heal. BC Canada: New Society Publishers. 2004.

www.greenfacts.org/en/endocrne-disruptors/endocrine-disruptors.htm

www.huffingtonpost.com/deborah-burnes/skin-care_b_1540929.html

www.organicconsumers.org/news/how-toxic-are-your-household-cleaning-supplies

www.theguardian.com/lifeandstyle/2015/apr/30/fda-cosmetics-health-nih-epa-environmental-working-group

www.webmed.com/asthma/news/20120307/study-links-common-household-products-asthma#3

"Young Living" Therapeutic Grade. http://www.youngliving.com/en_US/company/TherapeuticGrade.

LEARN MORE...

This is just the tip of the iceberg when it comes to all of the possibilities for using essential oils in your personal recipes. The oils mentioned are only a fraction of the collection. Talk to your local Young Living member about all of the collection as well as discounts and rewards for using Young Living products.

SHARE MORE...

Life Science Publishing and Products has everything you need to explore the history, the traditions, the research, the science, and the uses for all essential oils. Visit www.discoverlsp.com to learn how you can make the most of every essential oil single or blend. Whether you need books or tools for your home, glassware for your business, or brochures for helping you share, consider Life Science Publishing and Products your perfect partner.